THE SECRET TO HEALTHY SHINNING SKIN AT ANY AGE

MY STORY   WITH DRY SKIN

The skin is the mirror of your health

Take care of your skin, the biggest organ of your body.

BY   S. ELIA

The skin is the mirror of your health!

Self-published by S.ELIA

with the   Kindle Direct Publishing
@amazon.com

not for any medical advice . Should the reader needs expert advice ON ANYTHING, he or she should consult an expert of that field. If at any time you have a skin reaction from using any food , medication or other substance, you should consult your trusted doctor for proper diagnosis and treatment. Ultimately The reader is responsible for his or her choices , actions and decisions.

Table of contents

1)Introduction.

From time immemorial people are fascinated with a youthful , clear beautiful skin which is the personification of beauty. All people want to have a beautiful skin which is the essence of beauty and good health.
Some people, probably due to genetics, they have a natural beautiful, radiant , healthy skin , and

with the proper care they keep their beautiful healthy skin until they are old.

Some people are born with beautiful healthy skin but because of poor diets , the use of chemicals and not taking good care of their skin , they end up with bad skin conditions and spending a lot of money trying to restore their lost beauty.

The fact is, that most people, of all races when they are born and during their early years, have beautiful skin. But, as time goes by .nutrition, personal habits and the elements of nature have a dramatic effect on peoples **skin.**

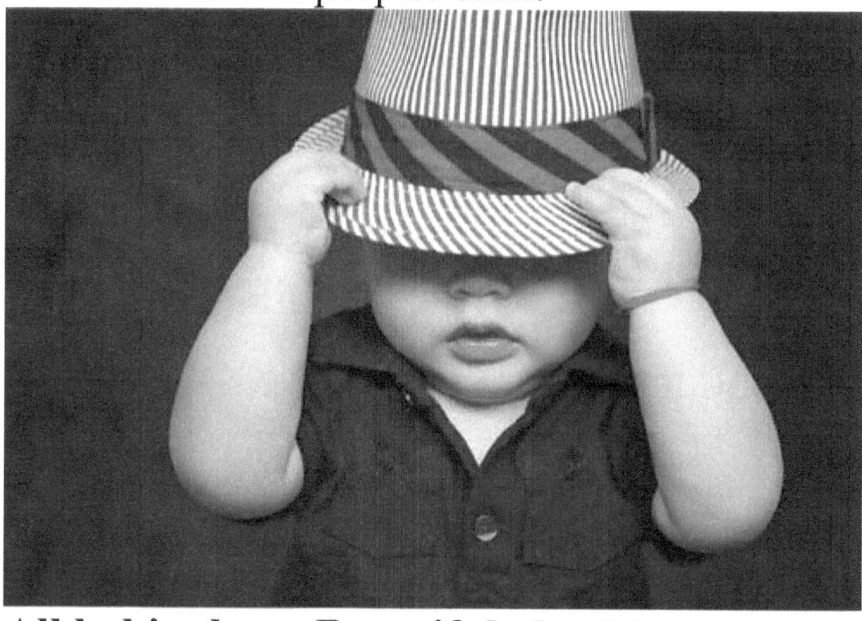

All babies have Beautiful, healthy, radiant skin .

The big secret of maintaining a youthful healthy and radiant skin is to avoid anything that has a detrimental effect on the health of the skin and the health of the whole body in general. It is not just your age that causes damage to your skin, it is the way you live and take care of your skin.

Things that have a dramatic effect on the skin's health ,are the effects of the elements of nature, the sun the wind, the cold, personal habits, nutrition, injuries to the skin , neglect, abuse and diseases. In this book we are going to examine the causes that are harming the skin and ways to avoid them and in the process to have a healthy radiant skin. I will start with my personal skin story and how I overcame the affliction of dry flaking skin.

2)My story

For years I was suffering from dry skin. Every summer my skin was damaging from the strong rays of the sun and was peeling off. With a slight rubbing of my forearms and you could see a lot of dead skin flakes falling off. There was no pain or anything just dead skin falling off. The same thing was happening during the winter time due to the dry conditions from the winter heating of the indoors.

Over the years I was using some lotions trying to control the flakes and protect my skin. That was only a temporary solution and my skin was not getting any better.

When I was in my twenties I got a severe case of dandruff on my scalp with severe itching and a lot of dead flakes falling off. I went to a dermatologist who diagnosed the problem as a severe case of dandruff and he gave me a prescription for some medications and shampoo. I was using the shampoos and the medications but I did not see much improvement. I saw another dermatologist who gave me other medications and shampoos but he told me that there is not much he can do about my dandruff and that I should not expect much. He was right . My dandruff continue to get worse and in a few years my thick glorious hair that was my pride and joy, covering my head , was gone and I ended up with a nice shining scalp . I was devastated. My hair was gone, and I ended up with a shinning bald head. The dandruff was still present and there were a lot of dead skin flaking off my shinning scalp.

I started using hats, and other head coverings when I was going out. I bought a hair piece to cover my bald head but I was not comfortable with it, as it was too hot in the summer time. I was seriously considering to have a hair transplant and I visited several doctors that they were specializing in that field. The last doctor I saw he had a bald head too, with very little hair on the side of his head. I asked him if he was considering having a hair transplant too, but he said that he was comfortable with his bald head and no, he was not going to have any hair transplants for his bald hair. He told me the cost of his services and he advised me to think about my hair transplantation and call him back to schedule for my procedure as there was a long waiting list for his services.

I went home and I was seriously thinking about his advice and the fact that he, a rich good looking doctor was comfortable with his bald head. I was also wondering how many other rich and famous people had bald heads and were ok with that.

Over the next few weeks I watch on television and the newspapers many rich and famous people with no hair and bald heads. There were even some famous people that they had hair but they chose to shave their hair off and have bald heads.

So I came to the conclusion that having a bald head without any hair is not that bad after all. If rich and famous people were comfortable with their bald heads ,why should I worry about the loss of my glorious hair? After all, In the long run , it would save me a lot of money for haircuts and other maintenance costs for my hair.

I called the doctor and told him that I change my mind and I was not interesting in hair plants any more. He told me , that's ok with him, and I if I ever change my mind, to call him back to schedule an appointment.

I put wigs and hairpieces away and started to enjoy my bald head. Feeling the fresh air on my bald head was refreshing. I even coined the phrase ," it is fashionable to be bald" and" bald is beautiful and sexy". I still had dandruff but I stopped paying any attention to that as I noticed that many other people had the same problem and they did not mind that at all.

As I mention above , I always had dry skin all over my body and flakes of dead skin accompanying me everywhere.

I thought that I was destined to live my life with flakes of dead skin to cover my place anywhere I was going. I came to the conclusion that it was part of my life, and I should be lucky that I had only flakes of dead skin and not something else worse than dry skin.

I recently read somewhere that scientists discovered that those flakes of dead skin are actually beneficial to the environment by reducing ozone or something.

Read this excerpt to see what they said , ""Flakes

of skin that people shed at the rate of 500 million cells every day are not just a nuisance — the source of dandruff, for instance, and a major contributor to house dust. They actually can be beneficial. A new study, published in the American Chemical Society's journal, *Environmental Science & Technology*, concludes that oil in those skin cells makes a small contribution to reducing indoor air pollution."

Now I do not know how all those flakes of dead skin can reduce pollution and how the scientists came to that conclusion, but I prefer rather not to have those annoying flakes of dead skin falling of my skin. I just mention it here and you draw your own conclusions whether those flake of dead skin are good or bad for the environment.

Well, I do not know what the scientist will think of next. I personally prefer not to have any dandruff, dry skin and flakes of dead skin everywhere. I prefer to have a healthy skin without those annoying flakes of dead skin flying everywhere.

Anyway, After many years of suffering from dry skin, I discovered that a cheap home ingredient could help my flaking skin from shedding all that dead skin cells. I used it on my arms and legs, and scalp and the dry skin, the flakes are gone for good. I said wow, why I did not know about this

stuff years ago? It could probably save my glorious hair. But even though my hair is gone, it is still my personal satisfaction to see my skin healthy without any flakes of dead skin flying all over the place and no more itching.
I found this cheap home ingredient to be very effective at controlling the flakes of dead skin and giving my skin a healthy shinning look. I use it everyday and I am sure I will use it forever.

After giving it a lot of thought ,I decided to write a book about my experience and the effect that a cheap home ingredient has on my skin , so that other people suffering from dry skin and shedding a lot of flakes of dead skin they will benefit from my personal experience. I hope that other people with this problem will have the same results and get rid of the annoying flakes of dead skin.

3) What is the skin

For humans, skin is the thin layer of tissue forming the natural outer covering of the body of a person or animal. When you look at your body you just see the exterior surface of your body , and that's your skin.

Of course there are other meanings when you hear the word skin but in this book we are talking about the thin protective layer that covers our bodies. Skin have all the living creatures including animals, humans which of course are animals too, the plants , even the plants 'fruits and seeds. No matter where you find the skin it is always for protection of the animals, humans plants and fruits. Without that protective layer of skin to hold everything in place, nothing can survive.

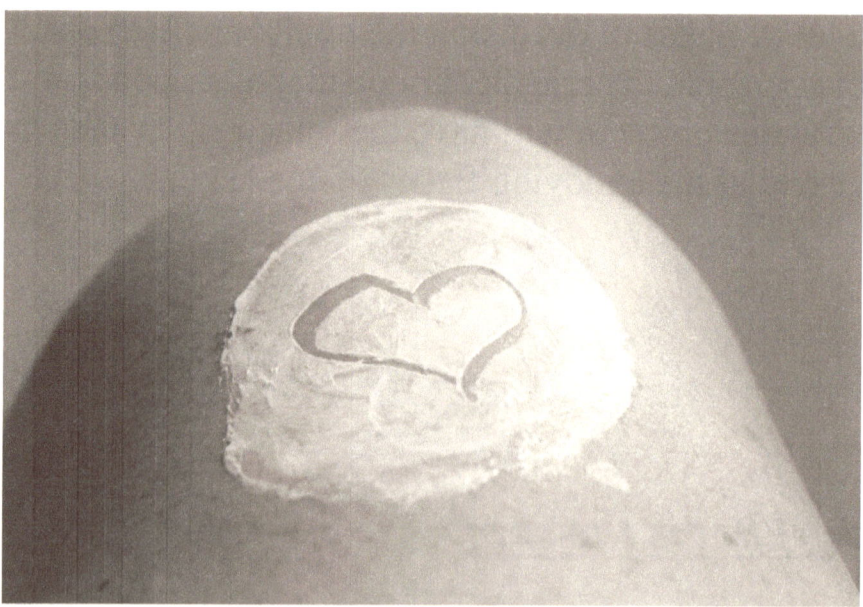

Picture of healthy skin

4) What is the purpose and function of the skin.

The skin is the biggest organ of the body and it covers the entire surface of the body..

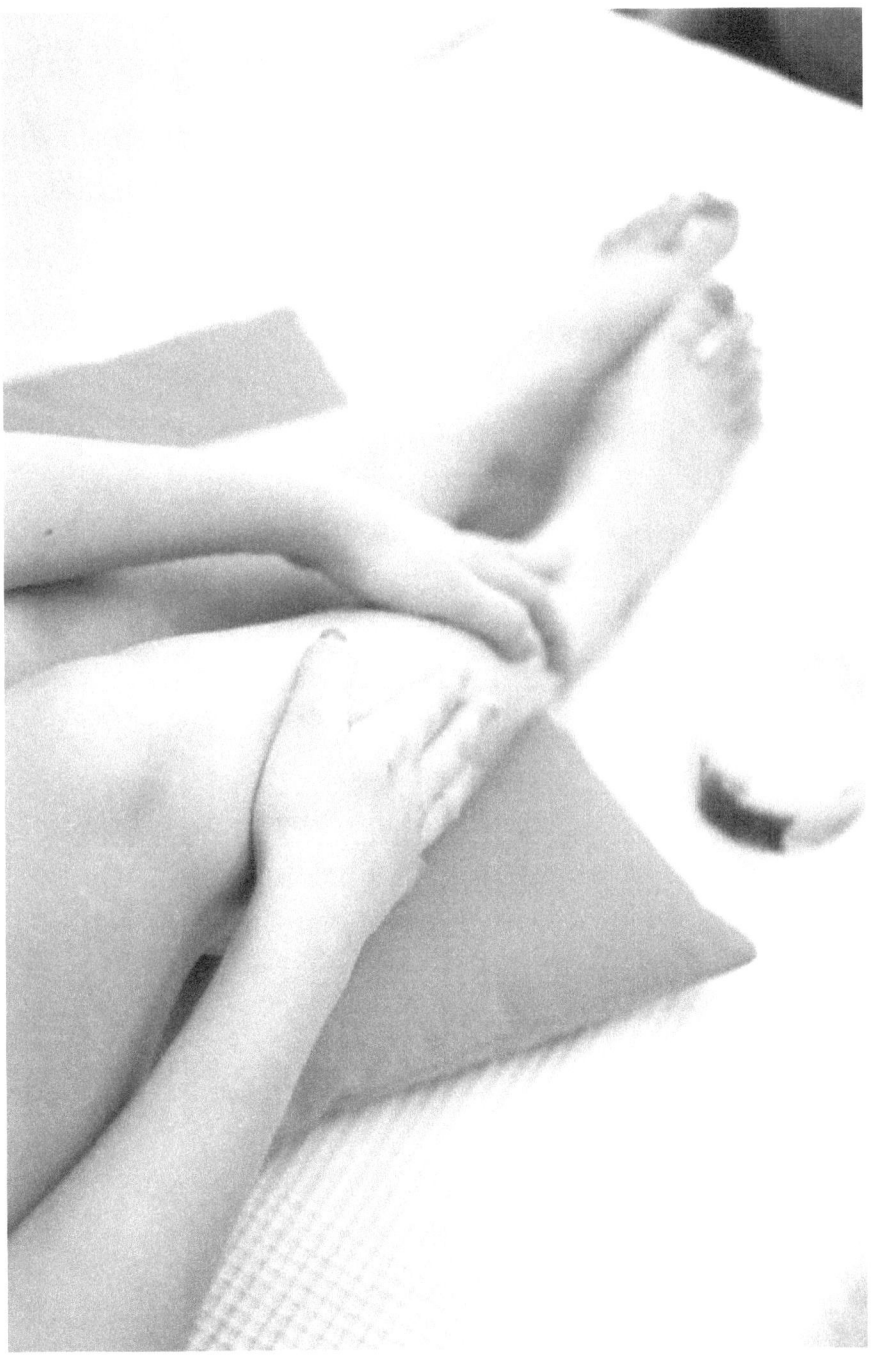

**The skin is very important for the survival of the human body.** Without the skin the human organism cannot survive. The survival rate for people with extensive injury to the skin depends on the amount of destruction of their skin surface. People with severe burns to their skin have a high incidence of non survival.

The skin covers the entire body and protects us from germs and the elements of nature. **It helps to regulate the body temperature**, and **permits the sensations of touch, heat, and cold**. The skin prevents any water or anything else to enter our bodies. The skin consists of two layers: the **epidermis and the dermis**. Beneath the dermis lies the hypodermis or subcutaneous fatty tissue for body insulation..

**The skin has three main functions: protection, regulation and sensation.** Wounding affects all the functions of the skin and can open the door for serious infections and diseases to the body.

5) The Skin has three layers:

a) *The epidermis*, which is the outer layer of skin, and it provides a waterproof barrier and creates our skin tone. Melanocytes are located in the epidermis and provide the color of the skin by producing the pigment melanin.

b) *The dermis*, beneath the epidermis, contains tough connective tissue, hair follicles, and sweat glands. The dermis plays a key role in Producing sweat and regulating the body's temperature. Within the dermis are sweat glands that produce sweat that comes out of the pores for cooling the skin surface when the temperature of the body is elevated from the normal temperature . It acts as the air-conditioning of the body. The layer of dermis is producing oil for the lubrication of the surface of the skin and preventing it from becoming dry. The sebaceous glands produce sebum or oil. Sebum prevents bacterial growth on the skin and conditions the hair and skin.

c)***The hypodermis*** , the deeper subcutaneous tissue is made of fat and connective tissue and it is mainly for body insulation and is commonly associated with obesity or being overweight. The hypodermis is prone to wrinkles, bags, and folds as the body ages that become evident on the outside. The hypodermis layer contains fat cells, connective tissue, larger nerves and blood vessels, and macrophages, cells which are part of the immune system and help protect the body from foreign intruders. Nature with all its wisdom provided everything for the protection of the body.

6)*Cleaning Your Skin*

It is very important to keep your skin clean to avoid any clogging of the skin pores to avoid infections and to feel fresh and clean.
Of course you have to wash your face every morning when you get up and any time you feel tired or sweating. It is not necessary to use soap, but if you have to use soap choose a mild soap

which does not cause any harm to the skin. If you want your skin to feel good and shiny , put a couple of drops of virgin olive oil in the palm of your hand, rub your palms together so that the oil covers the surface of both palms and gently apply it on your face. Rub your both palms with the olive oil and if you want , you can wipe the excess oil with a paper tissue. Do not wipe off the oil from your face. Leave it on your face and it will be absorbed by your skin and it will look and feel good.

If your skin is healthy, it is preferable that you do not use any make up that might cause a reaction or damage to your healthy skin, but of course that's a personal choice and you do what you want to do. For the rest of your skin you do not have to wash it every day , unless you sweat a lot. Take a bath or showers two three times a week will be plenty, unless you work out and you sweat a lot. Always use a mild soap on your skin . If you have dry flaking skin , put a few drops of olive oil in your palms and gently apply it on your skin. Your skin will absorb the olive oil and make it feel good, healthy and radiant.

Too much washing is not good for the skin as it washes the natural oils of the surface of the skin and makes it vulnerable injury and premature aging. If you have to wash your hands and skin often, it is a good idea to use a few drops of olive oil for protection.

7) Why is it important to have a healthy skin.

The skin is the mirror of your health.
 A healthy skin is an indication of good health.
A sick looking skin is an indication that the health
of that individual is not good.. The skin makes you
look and feel healthy, and beautiful , inspiring
confidence and feeling good. It makes a   good
first impression everywhere you go.
Having a healthy skin is an indication of good
health and the body is functioning properly.
A beautiful, smooth, youthful skin has positive
effects of well being that inspires confidence and
happiness. A healthy radiant skin is the desire of
young and old because it proclaims to the world
that you are healthy and beautiful.

8) The main functions of the skin are:

a) ***protection of the underlying tissues*** , keeping everything under control and keeping the body in optimum function.

b) ***sensational abilities*** to be able to feel the things you touch, the heat, the cold and pressure , and transfer that information to the brain for processing and the proper response. Nerve ending of the skin send messages to the brain about all the somatic senses including perception of pressure, heat, cold and pain.

c)***body heat regulation,*** controlling the body temperature and keeping the temperature constant for optimum body   function.

d)***excretion of harmful and waste products from the body, like toxins, salt and water.***

e)***secretion of oil to protect   the outer layers of the skin.***

The skin has **Sebaceous glands** that secrete an oily or waxy matter, called sebum, to lubricate and waterproof the skin and hair of mammals. In humans, the sebaceous glands occur in the greatest number on the face and scalp, but also on all parts of the skin except the palms of the hands and soles of the feet. Nature with all its wisdom, provides everything for the normal function and protection of the skin and the whole body.

f) ***absorption*** : the skin has the ability to absorb medications and other substances.

The skin when exposed to the sun rays produces the vitamin D which is very important to the human body for the regulation of calcium. Doctors have long known that vitamin D helps the body **absorb calcium** and is vital for strong, healthy bones. In fact, a lack of vitamin D can contribute to **weak bones** and fractures in people who have **osteoporosis**.

A healthy skin keeps the human body healthy. As we can see the skin has so many functions and it is very important and vital for normal function of the human body. So it is important to take good care of the skin and keep it healthy.

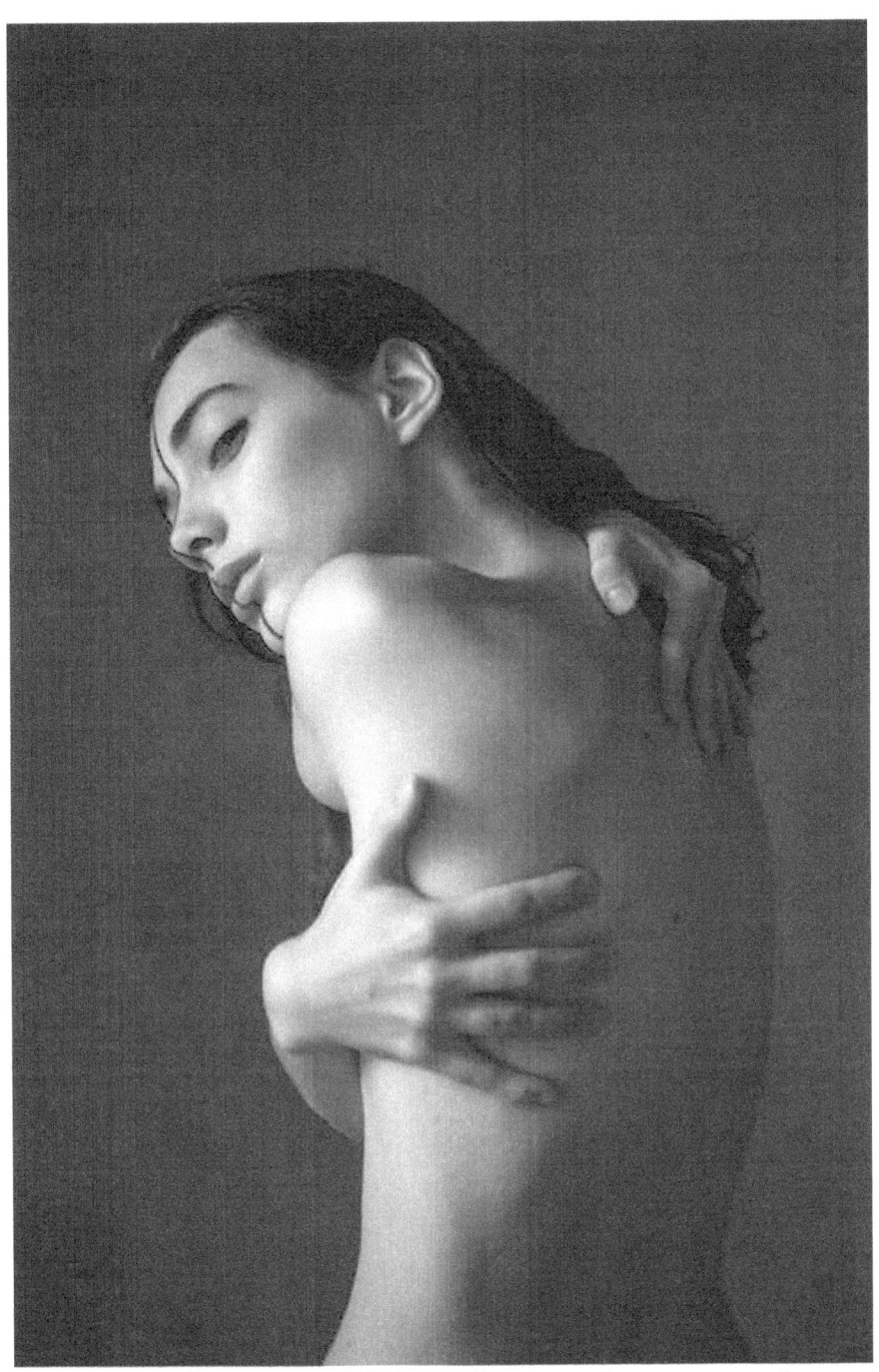

Healthy, clear youthful radiant and suntanned

skin that might be the admiration and envy of many.

9) In order to have healthy skin you have to Avoid the Things that can

damage the human skin

It is not only your age that causes damage to your skin, but the way you live your life and the way you treat or neglect your skin.
There are many **things** you **can** do to prevent the signs of aging, while there are also many **things** you may be doing that are damaging the health of your **skin.**

1) The number one enemy of the skin is excessive exposure to the sun rays.
Prolong exposure to the sun ages the skin prematurely and many times causes severe sunburns that can seriously damage the skin and cause skin scars.

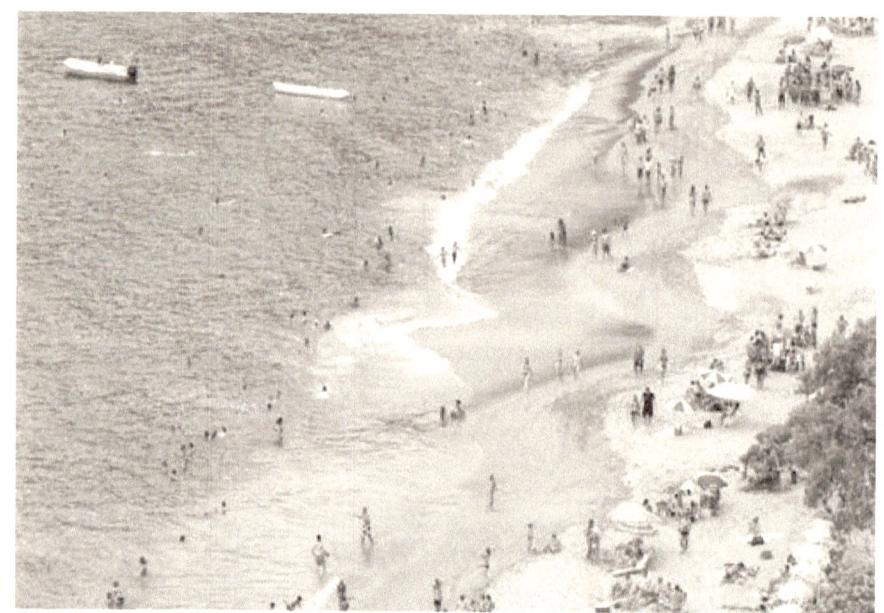

Natural sunlight, is also a skin cancer risk, sunburns, and other conditions. Limiting your exposure to the sun, can also help prevent wrinkles, dry and leathery skin, and freckles.

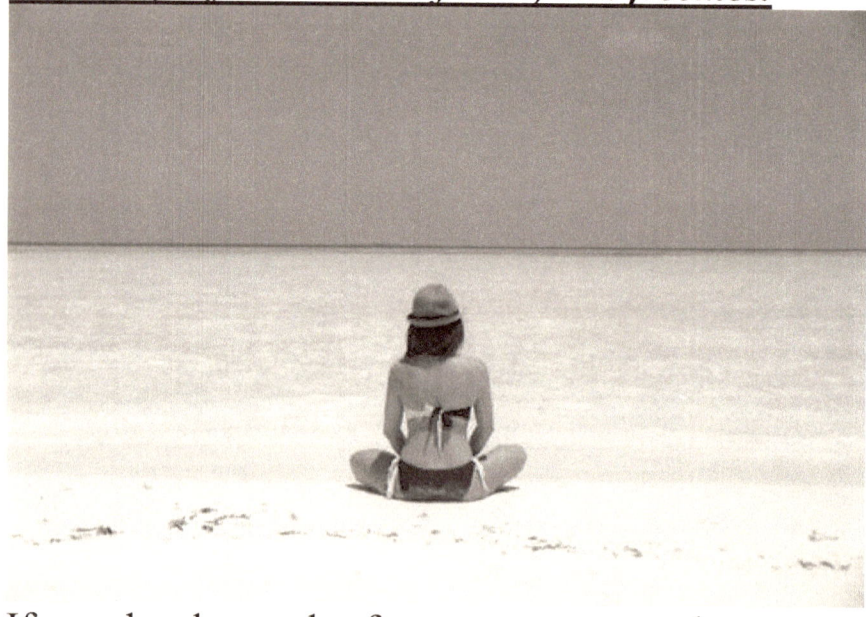

If you develop moles from sun exposure, be sure to

have them checked regularly if there are any changes in shape or color. Early detection of cancer can mean the difference between life and death.

2) _Excessive washing with strong soaps   washes away the natural oils of the skin and make it vulnerable   to dry and flaking skin which is the cause of many skin conditions._
Try to Limit bath time   and avoid strong soaps. Hot water and frequent long showers or baths remove the natural oils from your skin.

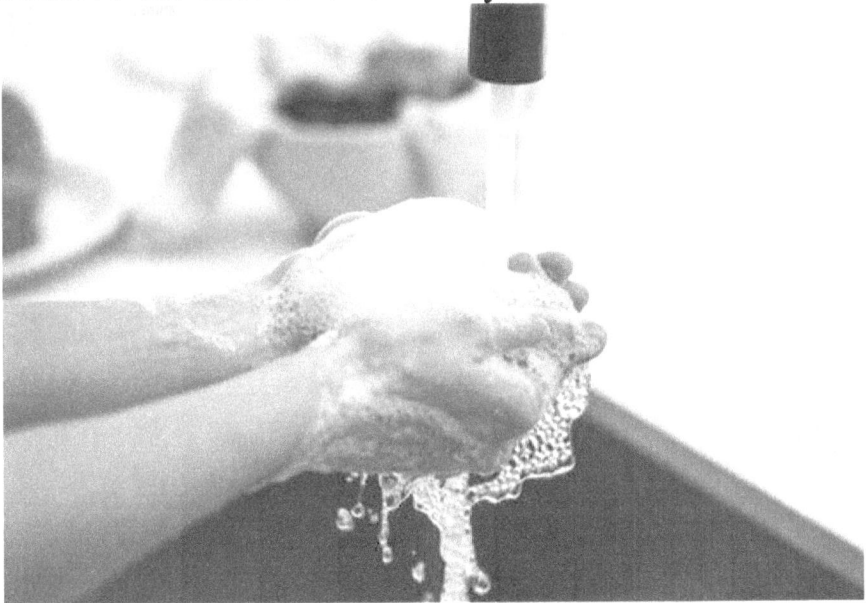

When you shave , apply shaving cream, lotion or gel before shaving To protect and lubricate your skin and Shave carefully.

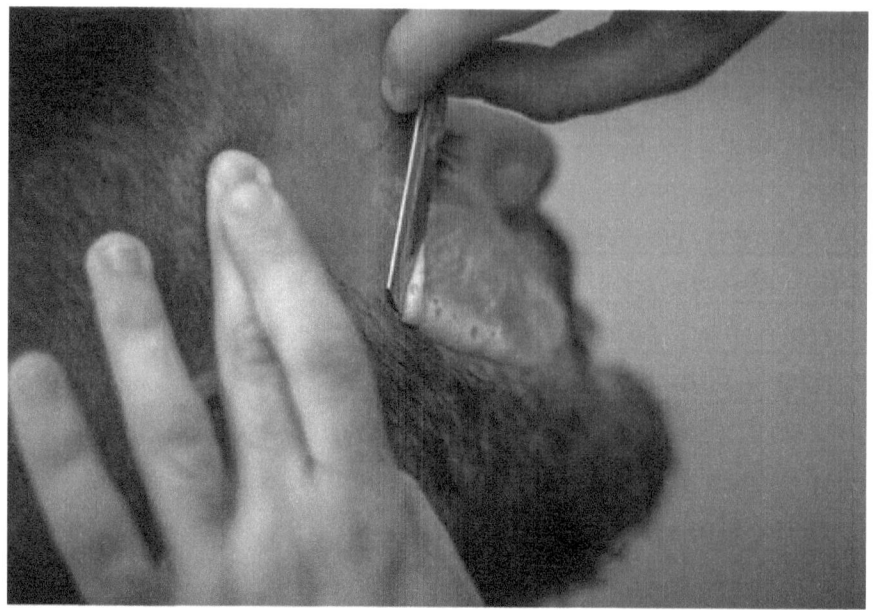

Any cuts or abrasions of the skin can be a source of infection and disease.

3) *Drinking alcohol and smoking causes damage to the skin.*

Smoking is proven to increase premature aging and wrinkles. You also increase your risk of skin and lung cancer. The damage caused by these habits may not show up right away but will gradually diminish the quality of your skin and health.

Try to quit smoking to prevent any damage to the health of your lungs and skin.

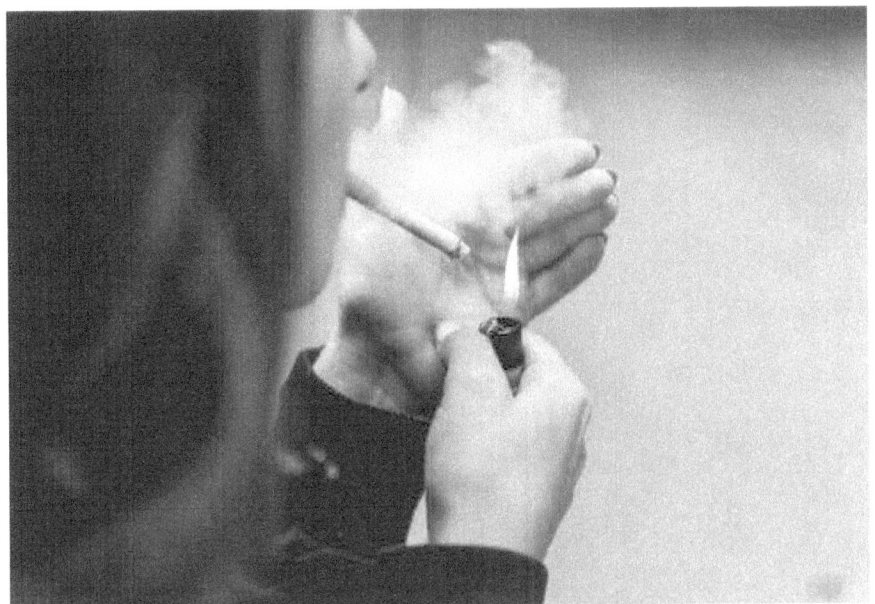

Smoking cigarettes isn't just bad for the inside of your body damaging your lungs and polluting your body with carbon dioxide and other pollutants in the cigarette smoke. It also pollutes the environment , the people around you, and it is bad for your looks by damaging the skin of your face with premature aging and wrinkles. And don't forget the damage to your hair and clothes that will have a bad smell of the cigarette smoke .

Stop drinking to protect your brain, your health and your skin.

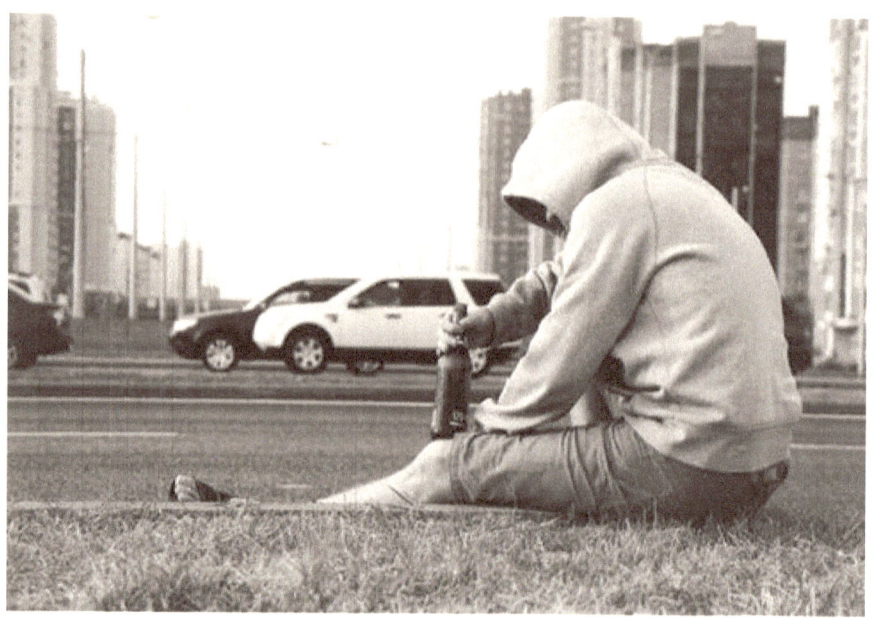

Drinking alcohol deprives the body of vitamins and minerals essential for good health and healthy skin, leading to malnutrition and diseases. Alcohol causes skin dehydration, blotchy redness of the skin and you can often tell a heavy drinker by the tone and color of his face. It can also cause dryness and puffiness of the skin and bruising and break outs due to malnutrition.

The American Academy of Family Physicians warns against excessive drinking when you are concerned about your skin . Alcohol can cause you to break out and have to deal with acne, whiteheads and other skin lesions. Excessive drinking may cause excess hormones in the body. Those hormones activate the sebaceous glands that cause your skin to overproduce oil on your skin, resulting in a broken out and pimply face.

If you want to have good health and a
healthy skin quit smoking and stop drinking.

4) _Chemical products_: your skin's worst
nightmare is when you use chemical based
products in attempt to keep your skin healthy and
young. If you don't get the desired results, you
keep shifting from one product to another and all
those chemical based products have a damaging
effect on the skin. These products are promoted as
make up for the face or body lotions and are
worldwide used by young and old people.

It is really frustrating and disheartening to see
young girls and others with natural healthy
beautiful skin using these chemical products
called, make up or body rubs and ending up with
all sorts of skin problems, allergies and other
conditions.

 If you are lucky enough to be blessed with natural
beautiful skin, count your blessings and avoid
heavy make ups to be more beautiful. Being
naturally beautiful is the best beauty of all, do not
mess up your beauty with expensive chemicals that
have the potential to damage your skin and end up

spending a lot of money trying to regain your lost beauty!

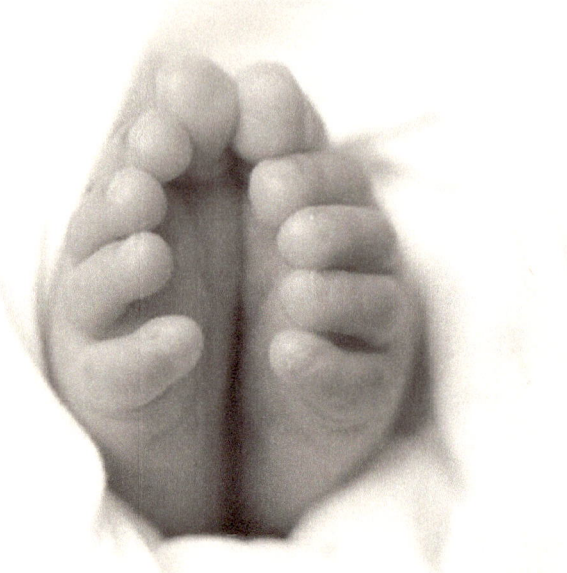

Beautiful healthy baby feet with radiant skin

A touch of a mild lipstick and a few drops of olive oil that's all you might need, and even that, use it only on special occasions. But then again, it is your skin, it is your face and it is your own decision what you want to do with it.

<u>5) *dehydration,*</u> : the human body is comprised of approximately 70 percent of water and it has a complex way of keeping the body water balance steady. When there is an imbalance it can cause dehydration or sealing of the body.

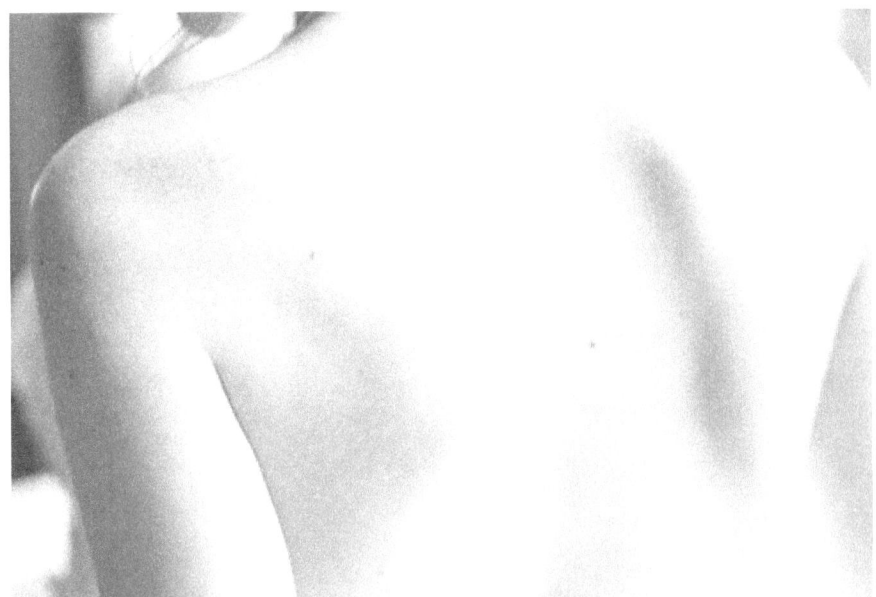

Dehydrated   and atrophied   skin, the signs of
malnourishment

The kidney, the lungs   and the sweat glands
excrete any excess water to keep the water balance
in the body. If you do not drink enough water, it
will result in dehydration dryness and a rough dull
skin.
You already know that water is the best friend for
your skin. It rejuvenates it from within by clearing
out harmful toxins from your body. Make it a habit
to drink

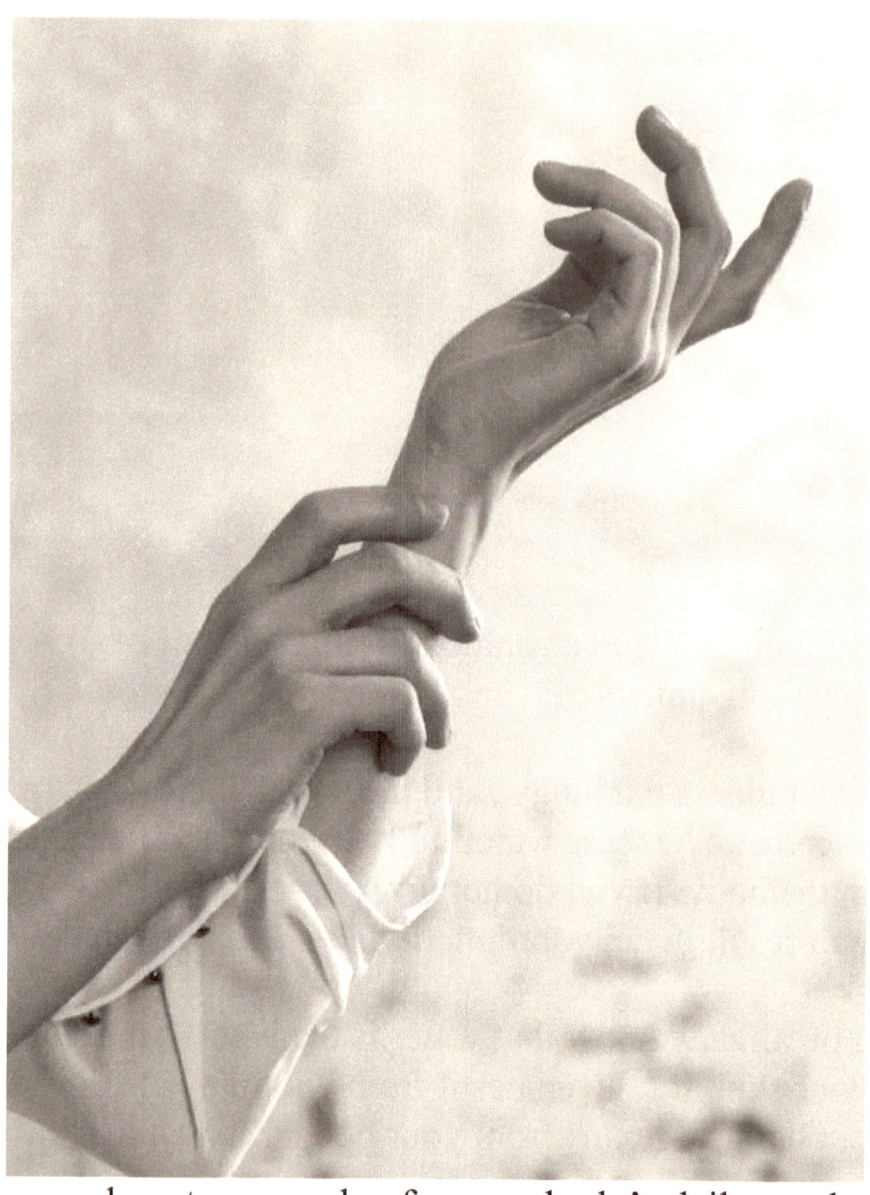

enough water everyday for your body's daily needs but never overdo it.

Moderation in all things as the old adage says.

Too much of anything can cause problems and that includes too much water.

Too much water in the body, It can even cause water poisoning and can result in death. There was a story in the newspapers of a water drinking competition, who can drink more water in the shortest period of time, and one of the contestants ended up dead .

So drink only when your body needs water with the longing of thirst.

6) Lack of proper rest and sleep.

Rest and sleep is essential for the body to function properly. Researchers found that those who didn't sleep well exhibited more signs of skin aging including wrinkles , pigmentation and reduced skin elasticity. The Effects of Sleep Deprivation cause tired and red eyes , bags under the eyes and wrinkled dehydrated skin. Prolonged lack of rest and sleep causes wrinkles and premature aging including premature skin aging. One study found that sleep deprivation disrupted the skin barrier function and this could trigger inflammatory disorders such as psoriasis, eczema and dermatitis.

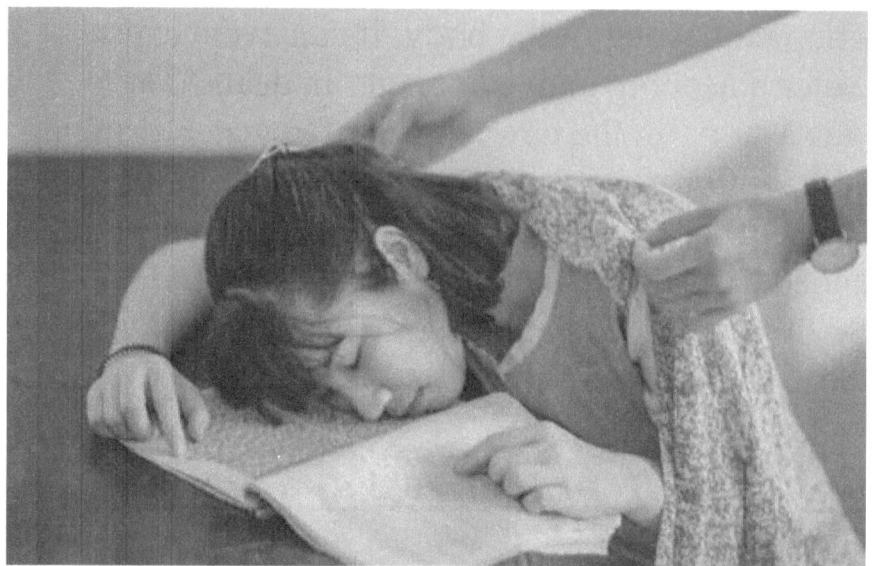

For good health and a healthy skin make sure you get enough rest and sleep everyday. Rest and sleep is the cornerstone of good health and vital for rejuvenation of the whole body including the biggest organ of the body, the skin.

7) the skin is affected by Nutritional deficiencies from bad eating habits, diets and hunger.

Nutritional deficiencies occur when people do not eat good nutritional foods or when they eat a lot of junk foods, ending up overfed and undernourished. The lack of the proper nutrition in the diet plays a huge role in the overall health and the first place to look for signs and clues is the skin.

In developed countries, vitamin and **nutritional deficiencies** most commonly result from poverty, restrictive diets, medication, alcoholism and inadequate dietary intake in the ill and elderly. Recognition of **skin** and nail changes can be an important tool for **diagnosing** underlying **nutritional deficiencies**.

With the nutritional deficiencies we have vitamin and mineral deficiencies which affect the health of skin and the whole body. These deficiencies can lead to many diseases of the major organs and the skin. People with anorexia nervosa starve their bodies from the required nutrients by refusing to eat .

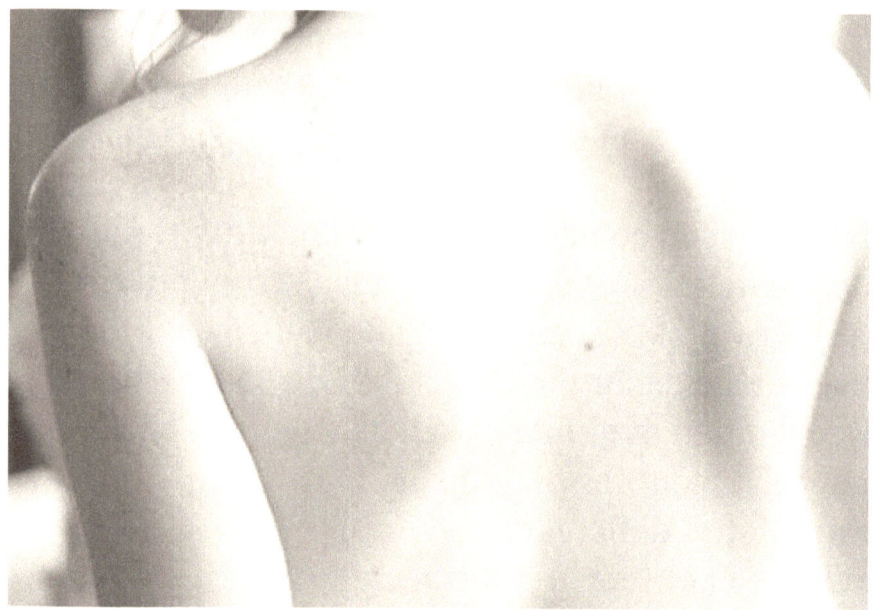

These people have an obsession to be thin and always think that they are overweight even when their body weight is malnourished and well underweight. These people and others that have nutritional vitamin and mineral deficiencies suffer from all sorts health problems and skin disorders. Some of their symptoms are, pale skin from iron deficiency, wasted muscles from protein deficiency, , easy bruising from vitamin C deficiency,, acne from vitamin A, E, C ,B 3, B6, biotin a zinc deficiency, scaly skin , horny skin, from Vitamins A, B2, and B7 deficiency. permanent goose-bumps, dermatitis , ridged nails and hair falling .

People with poor diets that eat over processed food with high calories and no nutritional values are also suffering from nutritional deficiencies.

They are overfed but undernourished and they suffer from many skin conditions and other maladies.
People on extreme diets are putting the health of their bodies in danger by not eating the right foods that provide the essential nutrients to the body. People on forced or voluntary hunger are in danger of developing serious diseases and even death if it lasts too long.

People suffering from the above nutritional deficiencies need to have a good nutritional diet and supplementation with the necessary vitamins and minerals. These people should be under the supervision of their trusted doctor for proper diagnosis and treatment of their predicament. Prevention is better than a cure. Having a nutritional diet and a daily multivitamin that works to keep your body stocked up with the nutrients it needs to function well will be extremely helpful in keeping your skin looking beautiful and functioning well.
And that is essential for your whole body.

8) dry environment

People living in cold climates are forced to have furnaces in their homes producing dry air heat, for heating. Dry air is the worst offender for the skin, taking moisture from the air and dehydrates the skin.. It simply sucks water from the skin, despite the skin's best attempts to keep it. It's a vicious cycle: When dry air takes moisture from our skin, its structure changes. Those changes make our skin less able to hold onto moisture and becomes dry and flaking with dead skin cells flying all over the place.

The only solution to fight the dry heat is to have a humidifier to

 Add moisture to the air. Even with humidifiers , it is difficult to control the moisture in   the house and sometimes it is too dry or too much moisture. As a result of this situation many people have problems with their skin, and sometimes it can even break up with deep fissures . Old people and people with health problems suffer more than others. Using various lotions and creams can help in a way with the dryness . Many retired people that can afford it , move in warmer climates like Florida and other warm destinations, during the winter and that is the best solution for them. Unfortunately not everybody can do that , and they have to stay in their homes and hope that the cold weather will be going away.   For all those people that suffer from dry skin during the cold winter months and the use of indoor heating, the best solution for them it would be to avoid taking too many showers or baths and use olive oil on their bodies to prevent dehydration and dry skin.   If they develop any skin cracks or fissures , they should seek expert medical help for the prevention and treatment of their skin condition.

9) direct and indirect injuries to the skin.

Any injuries to the skin from blunt or sharp instruments causes damage to the skin. Any accidental burns from fires can have devastated effects on the skin tissues.   Abnormal cold conditions can cause frostbites and destruction of the skin . If the damage of the frostbite injuries is severe it can cause the loss of the affected skin and even result in death.
It is very important to take good care of the skin that protects our bodies from any adverse conditions. Any accidental or intentional injuries to the skin, might have detrimental effect on the skin and the health of whole body.

10) make-up . Well this one is the most

common offender that damages the skin of many people, especially women's faces.
In their quest to look beautiful many women use make up on a daily basis. Some of them cover their entire face with various make-up , that all you see

is a painted face and no real skin exposure. Sometimes they overdo it and do not give a chance to their skin to breath. They put various creams as a night mask on their face. In the morning after they wash their face they put a moisturizing product on their face. Then they use a brush to apply the foundation all over their face skin and blend it onto the neck. Then they apply Concealer make up below the eyes in the shape of a triangle to draw attention to the eyes. that's a lot of work and a lot of expensive chemical products that affect the normal function of the skin.

As a result many people who use excessive make up they end up with skin problems as a reaction to all those chemicals that use to manufacture the make up products.

There is nothing wrong to use a kittle bit of make up, trying to look more beautiful when needed, but overdoing it has the opposite effect and causes damage to the skin .

I know it is your face and you can do what ever you want to it, but is it worth damaging your beautiful healthy skin by covering it with all that unnatural products ?

It is disheartening to see young beautiful faces and after using make up and other products on their faces in an attempt to look more beautiful, they end up with all sorts of problems on their faces' skin.

People, if you have a healthy beautiful face, count your blessings and do not destroy that beautiful skin of yours with chemicals that your face does not need.

If you really want to look beautiful, Just put a huge smile on that beautiful face of yours and that is the best make up you need to give your face a shining glow .

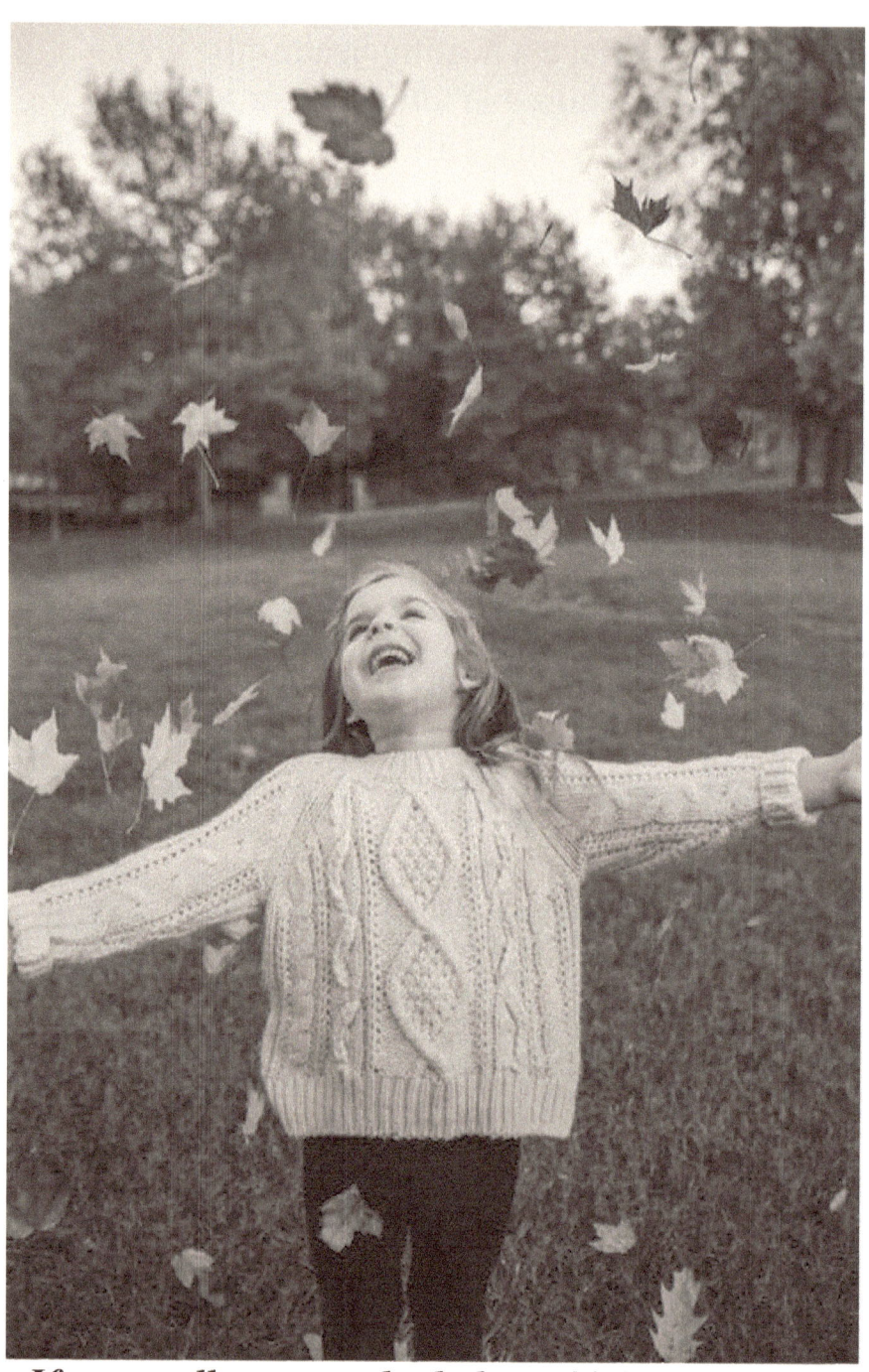

If you really want to look beautiful, Just put a

huge smile on that beautiful face of yours and
that is the best make up you need to give your
face   a shining glow .

'Legal Simplicity

All photos on Pexels can be used for free.
All pictures in this book are from the   Pexels website
Which according to their policy are "Free stock
photos you can use everywhere. **Free** for
commercial use No attribution required"

10) The benefits of a healthy skin

The benefits of a healthy skin is immense. It
makes you look and feel healthy, and beautiful ,
inspiring confidence and feeling good. It makes a
good first impression everywhere you go.
Having a healthy skin is an indication of good
health and the body is functioning properly. A
beautiful, smooth, youthful skin has positive
effects of well being that inspires confidence and
happiness. From time immemorial people liked to

have a beautiful healthy skin as an indication of good health and prosperity. In all nationalities and races, People measure beauty with the condition of the peoples skin . A clear, smooth , radian, shining , healthy skin is the epitome of beauty. They even name Aphrodite as the goddess of grace and beauty with that smooth healthy beautiful skin. Many women were famous for their beauty and their grace like queen Cleopatra and Helen of troy and because of her beauty caused the Trojan war.

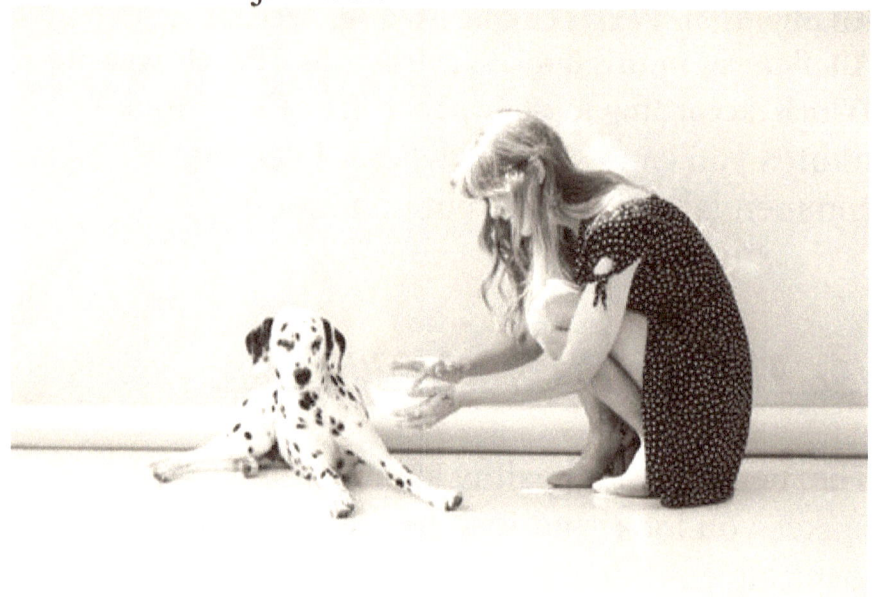

 A healthy skin will protect the body from infections and other diseases. By the same token, many diseases can affect the health of the skin. Allergies, liver disease, kidney and other internal organs diseases will have an effect on the skin.

that's why we say that the skin is the mirror of your health, a healthy skin equals to good health and a sick skin means a sick person.

The first thing we notice when we meet someone is the condition of their skin. If they have a healthy beautiful skin it makes a good first impression. Many great loves started from the first impression of their good healthy skin which we call beauty and instant attraction and love. If there is such thing as fountain of youth, then healthy skin care habits is one of it. A healthy skin keeps people looking younger of their age. it just feels so good when you face the world with a healthy and beautiful skin. It gives you an air of grace and self confidence . That is why so many women spend a vast amount money for skin products to make their skin look young and beautiful. It is essential to develop good and consistent habits when caring for your skin in order to make it glowing, radiant and youthful.

  Apart from that, having a healthy skin also means a healthy body and mind. That was the motto of ancient Greeks, that they spend a lot time exercising and treating their bodies to look beautiful both on the inside and the out side.

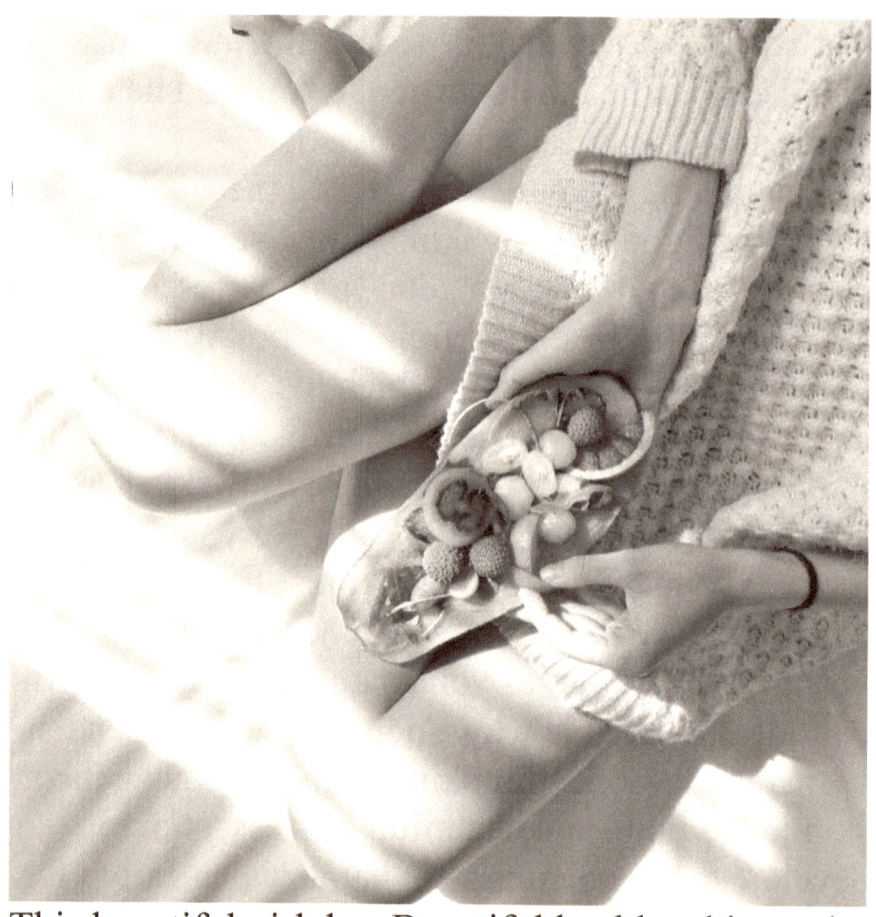

This beautiful girl has Beautiful healthy skin and she eats good nutritional fruits that provide vitamins and minerals for a radiant skin.

Kids have beautiful skin and they just look wonderful radiating with happiness , good health and joy. That would be wonderful if we could keep our youthful skin , but unfortunately we can not. But we should try to take care of our skin in order to combat these changes and keep our youthful look as long as possible..

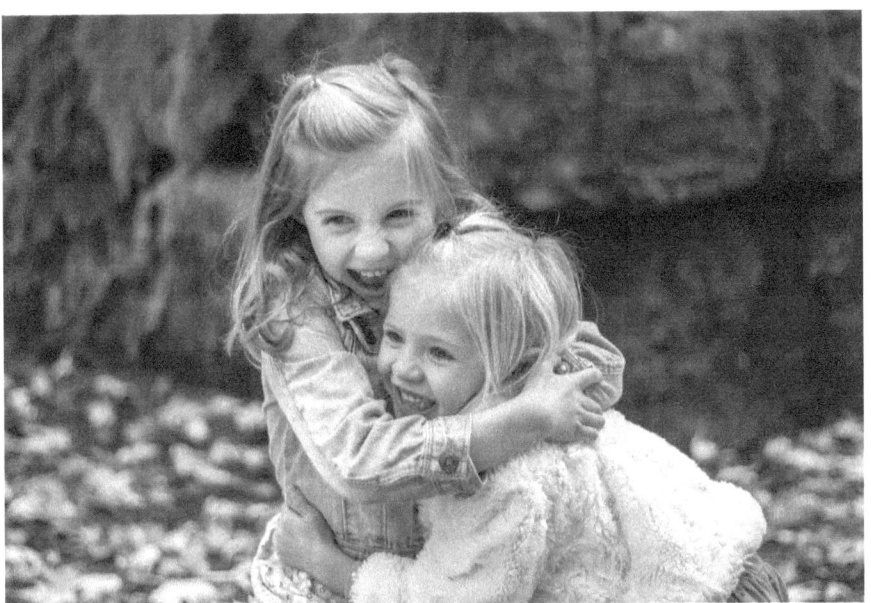

All kids have a healthy ,beautiful, radiant and
smooth skin which is the envy of many adults
with aging skin.

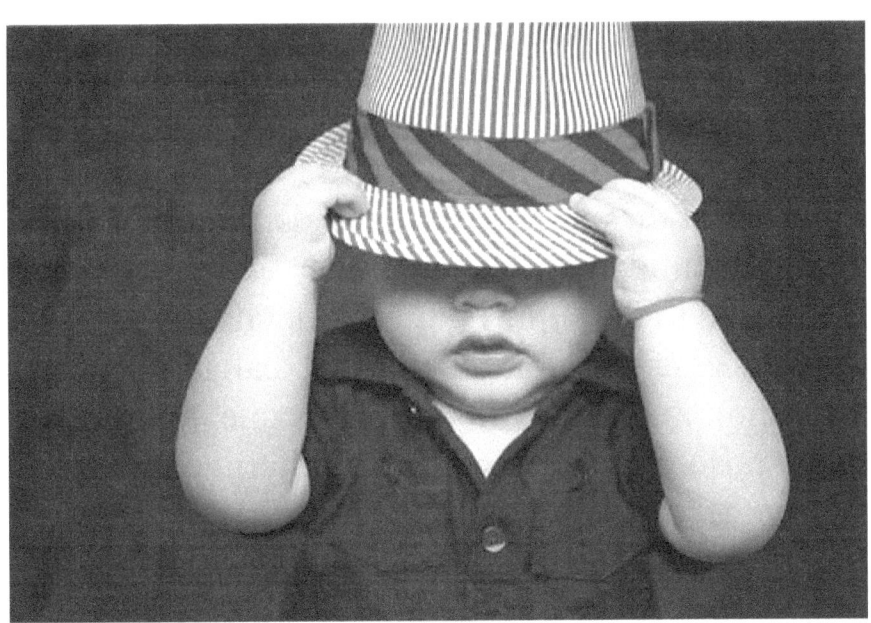

11) The secret for a healthy skin

The secret to have a beautiful healthy skin is to avoid what is causing damage to the skin. In other words you have to protect your skin from anything that can harm the skin .

As we mentioned previously the elements of nature has a detrimental effect on the skin.

Priority number one for a healthy skin is to avoid anything that has a negative and destructive effect on skin.

As we know, prolong exposure to the sun rays causes sunburns, destruction and premature aging of the skin. So it is imperative to limit the exposure to the sun for long periods and especially during the middle of the day. Since when the skin is exposed to the sunrays produces vitamin D, which is essential for the normal calcium regulation in the body, it is a preferable to have sun exposure in the morning and afternoon when the sun is not very strong.

In a nutshell , You should also avoid, smoking,

drinking or doing drugs which cause premature
aging of your skin.

You should avoid over washing your skin with strong soaps, which robs your skin of the protective oils of your skin.

You should try to avoid any injuries to your skin by using protective clothing and gloves when you work in your garden or anywhere else.

You should have enough rest and sleep to give your skin a chance to rest and rejuvenate.

You should drink enough water to keep your skin hydrated and avoid dehydration which causes premature aging.

You should avoid foods that have excessive salt and cured meat that have sodium nitrite or potassium nitrite which is bad for skin and your health.

You should avoid excessive make up on your face which   might not have the desired results you want, but on the contrary might cause damage to your healthy skin.

12)For healthy glowing skin you need a Good healthy diet with nutritional foods

You will also need to eat the right food to keep you in good shape.

There are many elements contributing to healthy radiant skin, including genetics, hormone balance,

skin care and nutrition. ***Food play a major role in the condition of the skin and without a proper, nutritional diet it is hard to achieve the perfect youthful healthy looking skin you want.***
You do not need a lot of money to buy expensive food to supply your body with the necessary nutrients. All you have to do is buy the right foodstuff at your local grocery chain and prepare it the proper way.

It is not the quantity of the food you eat but the quality of the food you eat that counts.
The right food will give your body the necessary nutrients to thrive! The wrong food in big quantities can make your body and mind sick and overweight. The Secret to Healthy Skin is the food you eat. A healthy diet which contains all the nutrients that your body need will do wonders for your body and your skin. We have all heard the phrase "we are what we eat" and we have to realize that this is actually very true and make it a habit to eat nutritional food for good health. By keeping constant healthy nutritional habits, the skin will be free from any of the dreaded skin diseases and conditions such as acne, inflammation, scarring, dermatitis, eczema, lupus, psoriasis and other conditions.

In a nutshell you should eat a balance diet to provide the needed nutrition for your body to function properly.

When your body has all the necessary nutrients your whole body will work like a well oiled machine and all the organs of the body , including the skin will thrive.
A balanced diet should include all the necessary protein needed by your body. Foods that contain proteins are the meats, eggs, milk, cheeses, fishes, grains and nuts and seeds.

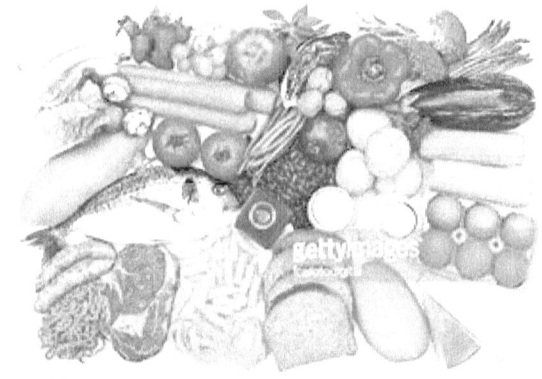

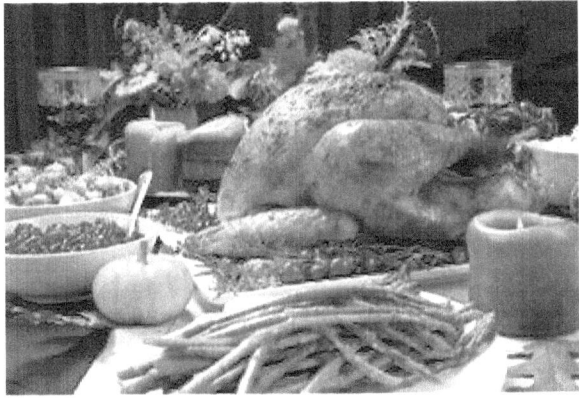
Proteins is essential for a healthy body and a perfect skin.

You should also eat a lot of fruits and vegetables which are the primary source of essential vitamins and minerals.

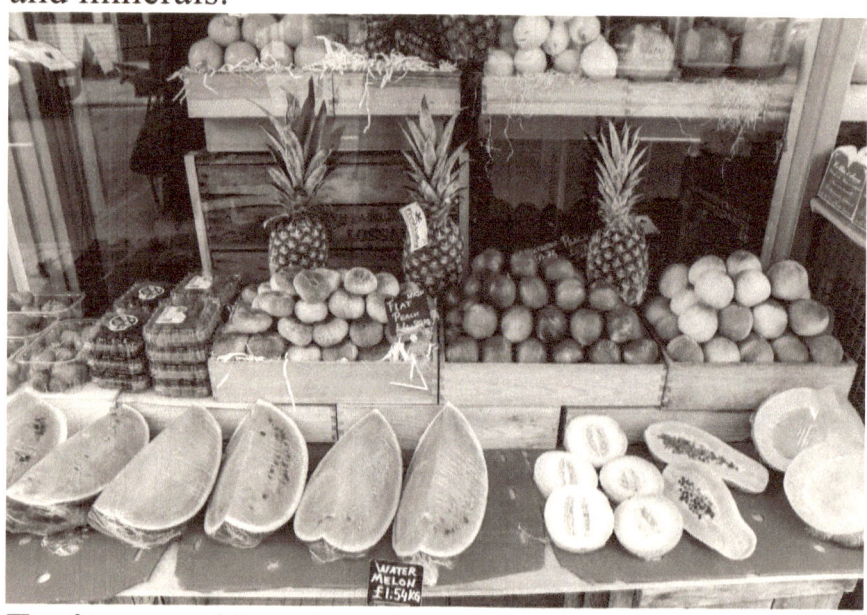

Fruits provide vitamins and minerals for a healthy body and

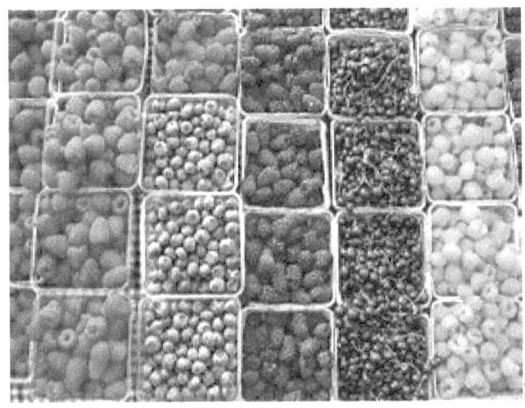skin. Vitamin C
and E are essential for healthy   skin.
The best foods to eat for a healthy youthful
radiant skin are fruits . Berries, fruits,
vegetables, Almonds, sunflower seeds, spinach,
avocado, sweet potato, wheat germ, dark leafy
greens, hazelnuts,   Carrot, squash, dark leafy
greens, sweet potato, pumpkin, red pepper, apricot,
mango, tomato, peach.
Whole grains, beans, legumes, nutritional yeast,
broccoli.
of course you do not have to eat all of them the
same day. You choose to eat the fruits and
vegetables you want every day. Choose to a
variety of fruits and change that variety often .
In a nutshell , lots of fruits and vegetables   provide
all the vitamins and minerals your body and skin
need .

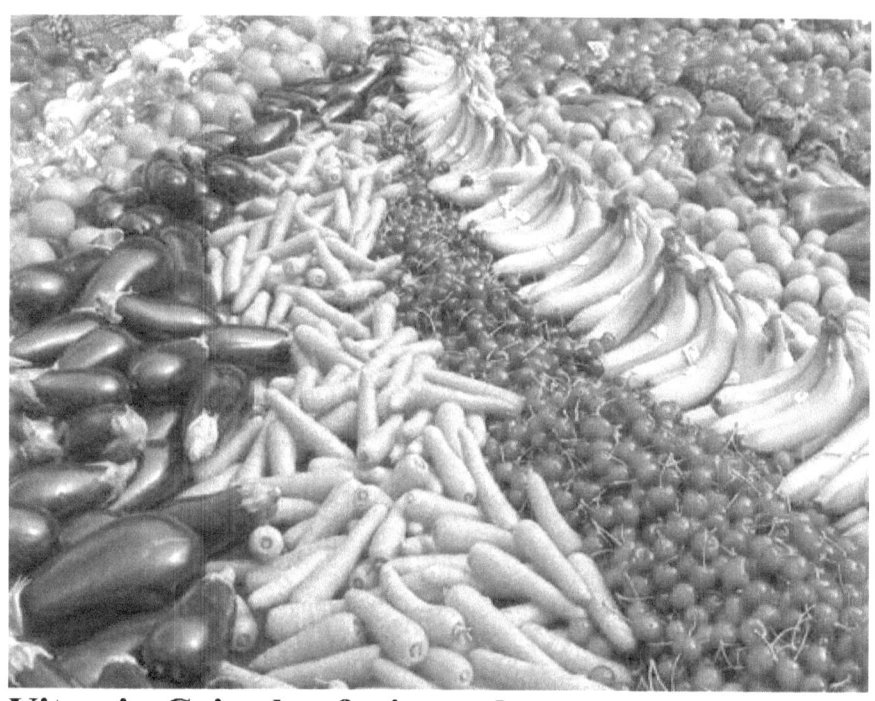

Vitamin C in the fruits and vegetables, promotes the skin-firming collagen in the dermis, and the prevention of dark spots on the skin. That is why you should eat vitamin C rich citrus fruits, leafy greens, berries, oranges and other citrus fruits, tomatoes, peas, peppers and other fruits and vegetables.

__Warning: some people are allergic to some foods or other substances and have a reaction to their skin .So anytime you eat something and you have a small or big reaction it is good to see your doctor for proper diagnosis and treatment. If you know that you are allergic to any food or any other substances, you should avoid those__

<u>*substances.*</u>

By avoiding everything that causes damage and
premature aging of your skin and eating a well
balance diet providing all the necessary nutritional
ingredients for your body, you will have   good
health and a healthy smoother, more radiant
young looking skin.
 It is essential to develop good nutritional health
habits when caring for your skin in order to make it
glowing, radiant and youthful

<u>13) The super secret for a glorious healthy young</u> <u>looking, radiant skin is   olive oil!</u>

 Well , well, well , this is the best kept secret
which is neither secret nor anything new. It is a
secret only for the people that do not know about
the health benefits of olive oil.
As I mentioned before I was suffering from dry
skin with shedding flaking dead skin from my
body especially my arms and legs.
 A few years ago, after working in my garden, my
dirty hands became dehydrated and stiff . So I
washed my hands with soap and warm water and
I applied   some olive oil on my hands to relieve
the dehydration and the stiffness . Because I

accidentally poured more olive in my palm than it was needed for rubbing my hands, I used the excess oil in my palms to rub my dry flaking forearms. I noticed that the olive oil on my forearms caused the skin to looked shiny, healthy and no flakes of dead skin were visible any more. I said , wow, that looks good, so I rubbed more olive oil on my dry flaking legs and feet. Again the dry flaking skin on my legs and feet looked better and the dead flaking skin cells almost disappear. I like that very much, and I thought that I was into something.

The next morning when I got up, I looked at my arms and legs and I noticed that my skin still looked good, better than before applying the olive oil the previous day, and less flakes of dead skin. My scalp was still covered with the flaking dead cells of skin.
I poured some olive oil in my palms and rubbed it on my scalp, arms and legs. Over the next few days I continued to rub olive oil on my scalp arms and legs and Lo and behold my skin looked good and I had no more dry flaking skin.
Ever since that accidental discovery, that olive oil was the perfect cure for my dry skin, I continue to use olive oil on my skin including my scalp. I have to say that I am impressed with the results and very pleased and happy that I got rid of my dry

skin and the annoying flakes of dead skin. Thinking that other people have the same problem with dry flaking skin and do not know what to do about it, I decided to write a book about my own experience with the olive oil and the pleasant results in getting rid of my flaking skin, hoping that my story will help them get rid of their dry flaking skin.

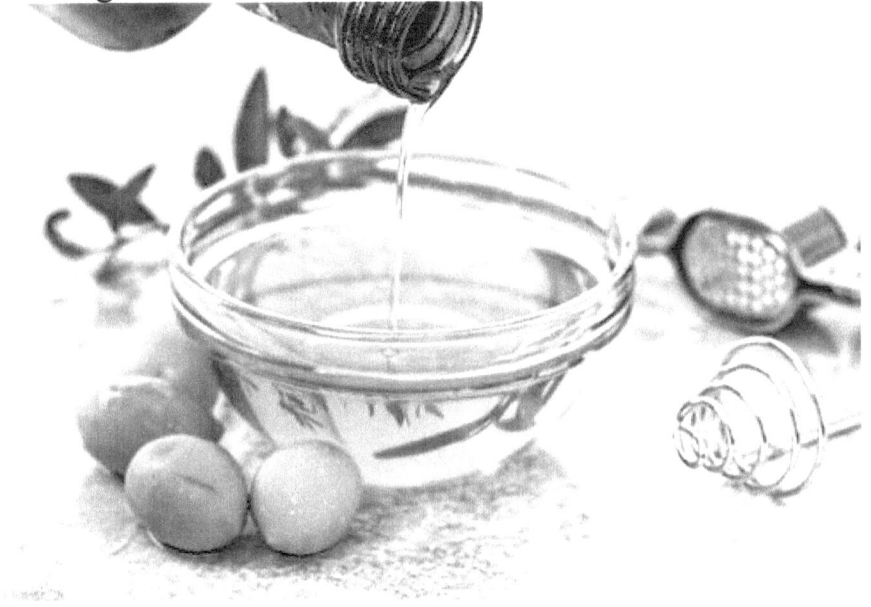

Olive oil is a good source of vitamin E and K ,which are both
important for cardiovascular health. Vitamin E is necessary to form red blood cells, and vitamin K is essential for normal blood clotting. Olive oil also contains small amounts of iron, calcium,

potassium and sodium.

A table spoon of olive oil provides 1.90 milligrams of vitamin E.

Vitamin E is the fertility vitamin.

Vitamin deficiencies that show up on your **skin** are **vitamin** A, D, C, E, B, B6, B12 in the form of rashes, flaky, dry **skin**, scaly **skin**, dermatitis, and white rashes.

Vitamin D is one of the best **vitamins** for your **skin**, along with **vitamins** C, E, and K. Making sure you get enough **vitamins** can keep your **skin** looking healthy and youthful

As I said above, the use of olive oil for good health and healthy skin, is neither a secret nor new. It is only a well kept secret from the people that do not know the health benefits of olive oil on the skin, and the whole body ,yet.

As a matter of fact, people have been using olive oil from time immemorial for many uses including for skin conditions.

In the bible You will find reference of using olive oil for the healing of wounds.

In ancient Greece, where they produce a lot of olive oil , they have been using olive oil in their daily diets , the so called " the Mediterranean diet," and for treating several conditions including skin conditions

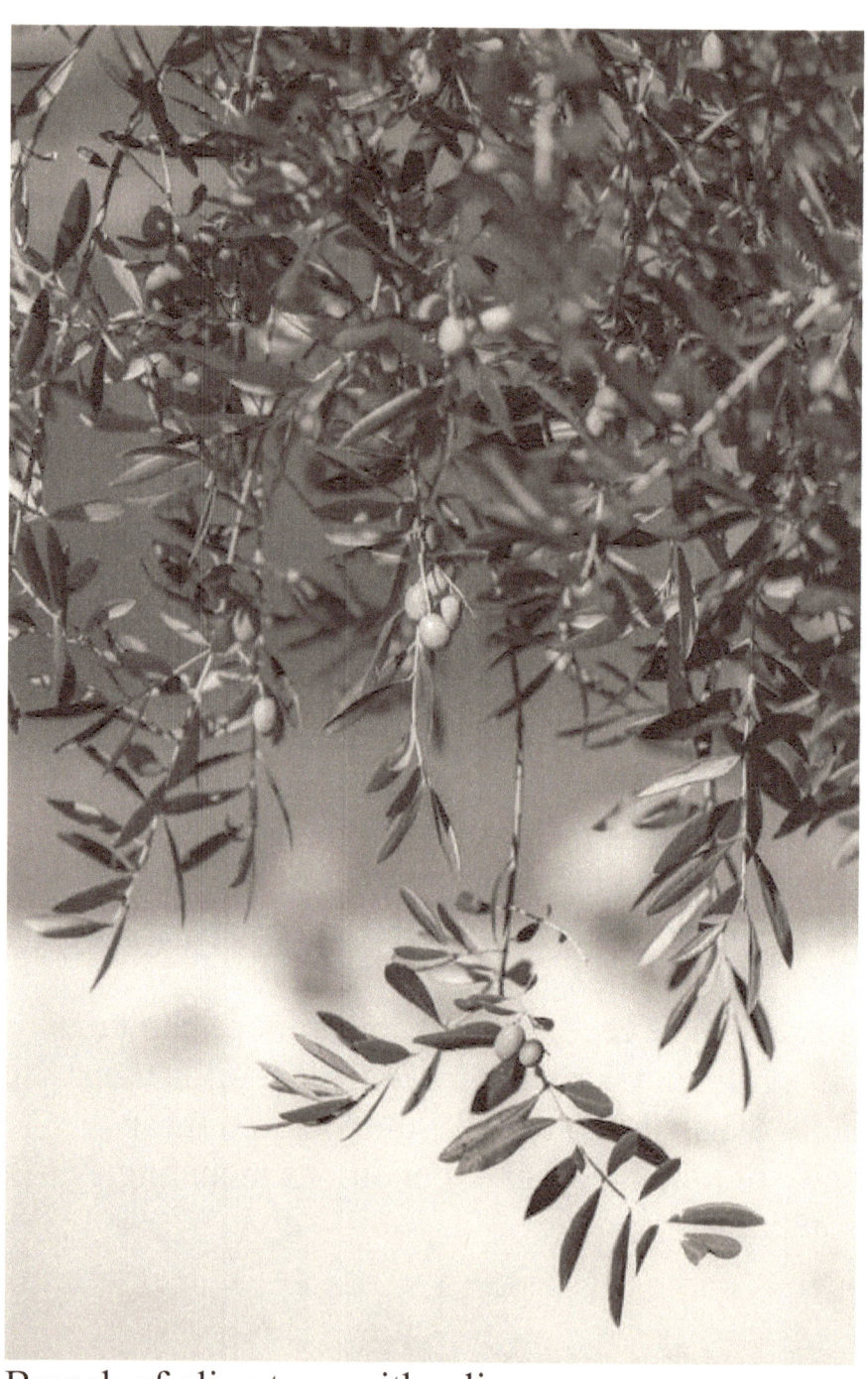

Branch of olive tree with olives.

Homer refers to the olive oil as the 'liquid gold'. Aristotle described the cultivation of olive trees as an important science.

Hippocrates, the father of medicine used olive oil to treat many conditions , including the healing of skin problems, stomach pains , ear infections and other conditions. Within the Hippocrates code, over sixty medical uses of olive oil can be found, the most common are mainly for healing of dermatological diseases. Also, olive oil is the base of the Hippocrates diet, in combination of course, with wine and bread. He also mentions that: "using oil in winter helps the body remain warm, because it stops the heat from escaping your body. And during the summer rub it on your body to nourish it and prevent overheating".

Solon made laws prohibiting to cut down or harm any olive tree.

The symbol of the olive tree has very deep roots in Greek tradition . It was the tree of peace and they pictured the Goddess of peace Irene with an olive branch placed in her hands. The olive tree symbolizes . Peace, wealth, health, wisdom and

abundance.   A branch of olive tree

and olives

The importance of olive oil has never faded and its nutritional and pharmaceutical value is now recognized

Greek athletes used to rub lots of olive oil on their skin . This natural oil kept their skin smooth, sensual, and appealing, and help regain elasticity of the athlete's muscles.

In France, Jeanne Louise Calment, the French woman , who lived to the ripe age of 122, credited Olive Oil with her youthful appearance and longevity.

14) The benefits of olive oil on your health and your skin.

Olive oil has been used by many cultures from time immemorial .

Olive oil is a liquid produced from olives, and it is a traditional tree crop of the Mediterranean Basin. The oil is produced by pressing whole green or black olives . It is commonly used in cooking, whether for frying or as a salad dressing. It is also used in pharmaceuticals, the production of soaps, and as a fuel for traditional oil lamps and in religious practices.

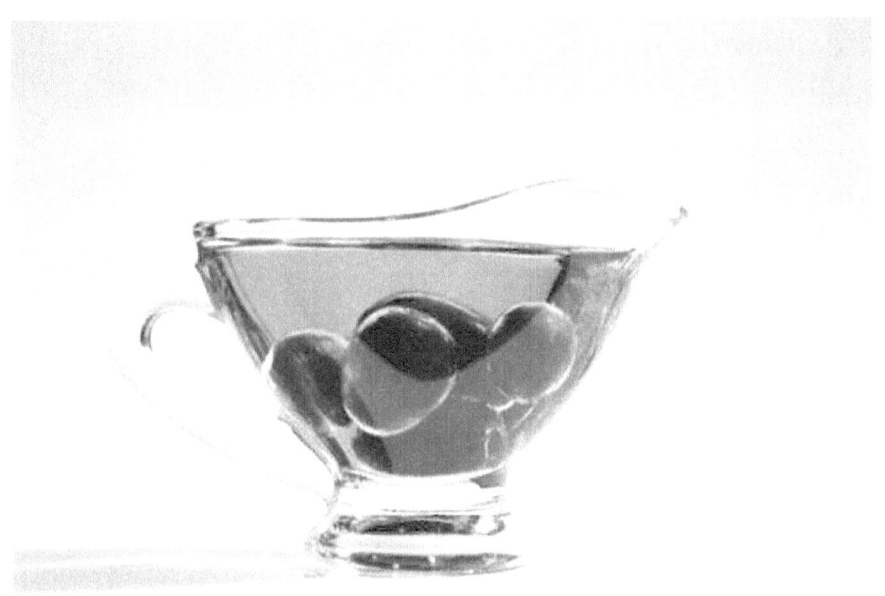

Olive oil can delay the aging process due to the high level of antioxidant content. Olive oil cleans, regenerates, softens and hydrates the skin and can help the skin regain elasticity. it can also help reduce hair loss .

Olive oil is a good source of vitamin E and K ,which are both

important for cardiovascular health. Vitamin E is necessary to form red blood cells, and vitamin K is essential for normal blood clotting. Olive oil also contains small amounts of iron, calcium, potassium and sodium.

A table spoon of olive oil provides 1.90 milligrams of vitamin E.

Vitamin E is the fertility vitamin.

Vitamin deficiencies that show up on your skin

are vitamin A, D, C, E, B, B6, B12 in the form of rashes, flaky, dry skin, scaly skin, dermatitis, and white rashes. Vitamin D is one of the best vitamins for your skin, along with vitamin C, E, and K. Making sure you get enough vitamins can keep your skin looking healthy and youthful

Olive oil boost the body metabolism, and brain function.
Improves hair health by supplying vitamin E and works as moisturizer of the skin and hair.
There are many claims about the magical healing properties of extra virgin oil , for preventing heart attacks, protecting the brain functions , promoting healing ,preventing hair loss and even preventing cancer and other conditions.
As far as I am concerned from personal experience, I got rid of my dry flaking skin by using olive oil on my skin daily. As far as the other claims, about the wonderful healing properties of olive oil, I have no personal knowledge or experience, but if there are claims by some people, it might be true. The fact is that it is a natural product and has been used for centuries by many cultures as food and medicinal use.

15)Who can expect to benefit from using olive oil?

I know that olive oil has helped me to get rid of my dry skin and all the dead flaking skin I had for years. But olive oil has a medicinal properties that can help many people with many other conditions of the skin and the body.

Here, I have to say that I do not endorse any brand or name of olive oil and I do not have any business or any other benefits , monetary or otherwise from promoting the olive oil use. I just tell my story how it happened to get rid of dry flaking skin by rubbing olive oil on my skin.

My purpose in writing this book is to help other people that have dry skin or any other condition for which olive oil might be beneficial.

I think that many people can benefit from using extra virgin oil either as food taking it internally with salads and other preparations of meals, or using it externally on their skin. Some people might make wild claims about some serious diseases that can be helped with olive oil, but , are these claims true? I have no idea.

The olive oil is a healthy product and it is good for daily use as food and as external application on the skin, but I have no idea if it can cure everything. Is it the elusive panacea? I have no idea but Time will tell ..

Anyway, olive oil withstood the test of time and it has been used from time immemorial by many cultures for their food needs, " the Mediterranean diet" and as an external rubbing on the skin for massages and skin conditions.

Olive oil has anti-aging properties and it is good to be used on the skin to prevent premature aging.. It also contains Vitamin B, D, and K and as well as Vitamin E that are more effective to your skin.

Vitamin E is the fertility vitamin and it might help improve the chances of pregnancy for women that have problems with fertility.

Olive oil might increase the virility and sexual endurance in men and women , as there are stories in some folklore that the women were advising their lovers to eat olive oil before visiting them for their sexual rendezvous. The Greek proverb , "φαε λαδι και ελα το βραδυ, " Eat olive oil and come over tonight " was their chant"

16) Try this recipe for fertility and virility.

In a bowl crack two large eggs and put one spoonful of extra virgin oil, mix it well and cook an omelet using olive oil in the heating pan.

Serve it with a salad of green leaves .

This recipe is good for women that want to conceive and men that want to be more virile.

Try it, you will enjoy it and it might be the answer

to your fertility and virility problems?…..NO
GUARANTEES.

Eggs have all the ingredients to form a new life, the chick, and are considered aphrodisiac .Olive oil contains vitamin E, the fertility vitamin and when you combine the two of them they can increase your libido and the chances of fertility.

People who live in dry areas can use olive oil to moisturize their skin and prevent dehydration and dry flaking skin.
Aging people face the risk of dry skin with fissures and opening wounds on the skin , the so called ulcers,, that might lead to infections . Daily application of virgin olive oil on their extremities will help the skin stay healthy and prevent any cracks on the skin.
Daily use of virgin olive on your skin might prevent the formation of wrinkles   and prevent dry aging skin.
For all those people that are blessed with natural beautiful skin, daily use of a few drops of olive oil will help them keep their beautiful skin healthy youthful and radiant. It will also save them a lot of money , as they will not need expensive make ups and the danger of damaging their skin from the chemicals in the make-ups. But again, people make their own decisions and they are responsible

for their own choices!
Olive oil can be used to revive dead or damaged skin and even used for protection from the rays of the sun. As we mention previously the sun is the number one enemy of the skin, so people should limit their exposure to the sun rays, especially around the noon hours.
Olive oil should be used in salads, in cooking and the Mediterranean diet for its health benefits.
The olive oil is the healthiest food containing powerful antioxidants and its daily use provides many health benefits on the whole human body including the skin.

17) If you have any skin condition

If you have any skin condition, please consult your dermatologist for proper diagnosis and treatment.
Many skin conditions might be the result of disease, allergy or other condition and you should let your doctor decide what is the best way to treat it. Nutritional deficiencies, infections and other conditions show up on the skin, and it is important to have a proper diagnosis and treatment. vitamin deficiencies that show up on your skin are vitamin A, D, C, E, B, B6, B12 in the form of rashes, flaky, dry scaly skin , dermatitis, and white rashes and

more.

Now if you get some small pimples try not to squeeze them as they contain pathogenic germs that can spread in other parts of your body. Just put a drop of iodine and a small bandage over and in a few days will go away.

If It is a big pimple do not bother it seek your doctors expert advice .

If you get an allergic reaction from eating something or coming in contact with something, seek medical help for proper diagnosis and treatment. Allergies is a serious problem that needs to be diagnosed and treated by the doctor.

18) Exercises

Your body needs exercises to stay in good shape.
Exercises increases the blood circulation in all parts of the body including the skin, and promotes the elimination of toxins and other waste products from the body. In short, exercises rejuvenate your skin and makes it look beautiful and healthy. Keep your workouts short and sweaty and you'll reap all the benefits of good health and a healthy glowing skin.

After your exercises and you have a shower, Applying olive oil on your skin and joints , will make your skin feel good, relaxed and radiant.
You do not need to spend a lot of money for gyms or expensive equipments.

A brisk walk around the block will do wonders to your body.
You can play, volley ball with your friends, or on the wall of your house if nobody else is available.
You can play with a bouncing ball for 15-20 minutes.
Swimming is excellent so are so many other sports you might like.
The idea is to exercise your body muscles and strong muscles usually have healthy beautiful skin.

You can exercise in the privacy of your home and even in your own bed for 20 to 30 minutes daily. You can find spinal exercises you can do at home which are good for exercising your spine for good health in my book : EUREKA: THE MOTHER CAUSE OF SCOLIOSIS. Available @ amazon.com

People that exercise regularly have good health a healthy youthful skin. Make it a habit to exercise regularly for the improvement of your health and your skin.

Jeanne Louise Calment, the French woman , who lived to the ripe age of 122 credited her longevity to her physical active live. She rode a bicycle every day until she turned 100 years old and she was also active with roller skating, tennis, hunting, and swimming. She had a healthy diet with the use of lots of olive oil, which she also used it on her skin daily.

The objective is not to live 122 years, but with exercises, good diet and the use of olive oil , your health and your skin will benefit tremendously.

19) Conclusion

The condition of your skin is the mirror of the condition of your body . It is essential to develop good and consistent habits when caring for your skin in order to make it glowing, radiant and youthful.

By avoiding everything that causes damage and premature aging to your skin and eating a well balance diet that provides all the necessary nutritional ingredients for your body, you will have good health and a healthy smoother, radiant young looking skin. In order to have healthy youthful radiant skin, you have to avoid the things that cause damage to the skin. All the things we mention above . Avoid excessive sun exposure, the cold , the wind, smoking , drinking, heavy make-up, , injuries to the skin, excessive washing with strong soaps, luck of rest and sleep, and anything that has a detrimental effect on the skin. It is also very important to have good nutrition for your body's nutritional needs. When your body has all the needed nutrients it will have an effect on your skin and having a healthy skin also means a healthy body and mind.

The health of your skin is the mirror of your body's health.

You should also exercises regularly to keep the tone of your skin healthy and to promote the elimination of waste and toxins from your body. A healthy body will have a healthy skin. It is as simple as that.

Eating healthier, exercising daily and working

towards a life of healthy skin while you're young , it will help your skin stay healthy into your golden years.
 Finally keep your skin clean and use a few drops of virgin olive to rub on your face and on your whole body skin , but particularly your arms and legs to make it feel good, healthy and radiant.
 Olive oil is a natural product which you can find in almost every kitchen. Many people use it daily for cooking, in salads and it is good to use it externally on your skin for protection and to make it shine.

   You will be surprised how good your skin will look and feel naturally.
To conclude , the secret to healthy youthful skin, is to avoid what harms the skin, exercise for strong healthy muscles and skin, eat a nutritional diet that provides all the nutrients needed for good healthy body and skin and finally the use of olive oil for protection and moisturizing.

20) References:
Photo Credits

Legal Simplicity

21) From The Author:

 The author is a retired health professional
interested in health issues, fitness, exercises,
nutrition and other lifestyle topics.
In this book he writes about his own story how he
overcame his condition of dry skin , with the hope
that his readers will have the same satisfactory
results as he did   and get rid of their dry skin.

22) Book description

This book is about my personal experience how I overcame my dry flaking skin.
Read this book to learn how to get rid of your dry flaking skin.
Read this book to learn about a cheap substance that can help you with your skin problems.
Read this book to learn how to improve your diet for better health and healthy skin.
In this book you will find what damages your skin.
In this book how to avoid the things that cause damage to your skin.
In this book you will find the recipe for fertility and virility. Try this cheap recipe for fertility and virility. it might improve your fertility and your virility.
In this book you will learn about a household

food that can help you achieve good health and healthy skin.

Just read this book out of curiosity about the best kept secret for healthier skin.

From the inside cover.

After reading this book and you no longer need it, give it to someone else to benefit from the knowledge in this book.

Knowledge is to be shared for the benefit all, and that is the main reason for witting books: to convey information.

If you find the knowledge in this book helpful for your skin problem, write a good review of this book, or recommend it to others.

www.ingramcontent.com/pod-product-compliance
Lightning Source LLC
Chambersburg PA
CBHW020605220526
45463CB00006B/2457